30 Day Rehab for Trichotill

Overcome Trichotillomania
How to Stop Hair pulling Disorder

Copyright © 2013 Sabrina Kendall - All Rights Reserved

Introduction

Thank you for your interest in this book. This is the beginning to your recovery of trichotillomania. You can stop hair pulling, this is a behavioral habit that many people have, but they hide it of course. The people that have trichotillomania think they are the only one, or they are part of a few people that pull their own hair out. There are hundreds maybe thousands of people that have trichotillomania.

Trichotillomania doesn't discriminate; children have it, teens, adults, Caucasian people, Koreans, African Americans, Latino Americans, Native Americans, etc.

I started pulling my hair out 10 years ago, so basically I've had trichotillomania for a decade. My family and other people that know me consider me to be intelligent; I will still accept that they say I'm smart. Although I pulled my hair for 10 years, I will not feel guilty or less intelligent.

Trichotillomania is a behavioral habit that can cause individuals to think negative thoughts about themselves and others; it's called "Obsessive Thoughts." Those continuous awful thoughts can make a person with trichotillomania feel sad, anxious, guilty, etc.

When you catch yourself having negative repetitive

obsessive thoughts, replace those thoughts with positive thoughts. Negative thoughts make people with health conditions and disorders get worse. Positive thoughts are known for making people with health conditions and disorders overcome their sickness.

When I first starting pulling my hair out, I was looking for other people to make me happy. I didn't have many hobbies to keep myself busy, and I was unemployed. I no longer look for others to make me happy, I choose to be happy own my own and when I'm alone. But people can add to my joy and happiness, I finally get it now.

A few nights I prayed to the Heavenly Father to bless me with new hobbies, to keep my hands busy in a constructive way instead of destructive with the hair pulling. Ten years ago when I pulled that first strand of hair, I didn't know that I was beginning to make a bad habit. Actually I didn't even know the name of the hair pulling condition, until I Google'd it on my computer 3 years into it.

When you believe you are healed and take action toward your healing, you will overcome trichotillomania. I'm a believer that all things are possible to them that believe; you can overcome trichotillomania when you believe you can. Christ Jesus is the healer.

If you find this book to be useful, please leave a positive comment in the review area of the Amazon page where this book is listed. Your positive comment will help others that are interested in overcoming trichotillomania, by starting a 30 rehab challenge as well. The 30 days is a start, fighting the itchy scalp urges to pull, may be a longer challenge. And you can stop responding to the urges to pull, it will take time.

Thank you.

Available Book Formats

This book is also available in an eBook format on Amazon's Kindle at ASIN: http://www.amazon.com/dp/B00HCLSD0E – you don't have to own a Kindle device to download an eBook, you can use a computer or other electronic computer device as well.

And available in audio-book format at ASIN: B00HYMQ6AK on Amazon.

I recommend that you purchase this book in all 3 formats, it will be helpful for your recovery of trichotillomania.

30 Day Rehab Challenge for Trichotillomania
copyright © 2014 by Sabrina Kendall

All rights reserved. No part of this book may be reproduced in any form without permission in writing from the author. Reviewers may quote brief passages in reviews.

Legal Disclaimer

No part of this publication may be reproduced or transmitted in any form or by any means, mechanical or electronic, including photocopying or recording, or by any information storage and retrieval system, or transmitted by email without permission in writing from the publisher.

While all attempts have been made to verify the information provided in this publication, the author does not assume any responsibility for errors, omissions, or contrary interpretations of the subject matter herein.

This book is for educational purposes only. The views expressed are those of the author alone, and should not be taken as expert instruction or commands. The reader is responsible for his or her own actions. Adherence to all applicable laws and regulations, including international, federal, state, and local governing professional licensing, business practices, advertising, and all other aspects of doing business in the US, Canada, or any other jurisdiction is the sole responsibility of the purchaser or reader. The author does not assume any responsibility or liability whatsoever on the behalf of the purchaser or reader of this book.

Thank you.

Copyright © 2013 Sabrina Kendall - All Rights Reserved

Contents

Introduction

Define Trichotillomania   1

Things to Avoid   3

What is OCD Obsessive Compulsive Disorder?   4

Symptoms of Trichotillomania 6

OCD Quiz for Trichotillomania 11

How to Stop Pulling Hair Out   15

30 Day Challenge   23

Define Trichotillomania

Trichotillomania is a nervous impulse that causes an individual to pull out their hair. Trichotillomania can be connected to having negative obsessive thoughts, usually negative thoughts or other related thoughts that may cause anxiety. This also can lead back to the behavioral habit called trichotillomania, commonly known as an obsessive compulsive disorder. This obsessive disorder causes short hair and/or bald spots on the head, due to repetitive hair pulling of one's own hair.

Trichotillomania often causes some people to pull because they first feel the urge to scratch their scalp, due to it being itchy from their OCD impulses. This can trick you into to pulling in that same spot where it itches.

Some people pull hair out when being tensed, and they may think after pulling they feel less tensed. In actuality the pulling is not making them less tensed or less anxious. The hair pulling is making the heart rate go up, and it's making the breathing pattern kind of off.

There are some people that say trichotillomania is a mental disorder, it's not a mental disorder. It's a behavioral disorder that's connecting with OCD nervous impulses.

30 Day Rehab Challenge for Trichotillomania 1

A hair puller can change the channel in their mind by exercising constructive and positive thinking patterns. Although it all starts in the mind, where the mind is, the body will follow.

"Trich"otillomania sometimes "trick" patients into a chain of other OCD behavior such as skin picking, eating the hair that's pulled out, continuous depressive thoughts, becoming less out-going, feeling guilty than usual, etc.

This hair-pulling disorder affects men, women, and children. Most people that pull notices at that moment, the feeling and thoughts their having are either sleepiness, tiredness, anxiety, hungry, bored, stress, or something else related to those. When having the feeling of sleepy in the day time it's better to take a 15 minute or more nap if possible.

Avoid letting trichotillomania take the place of you getting your rest or proper sleep. Trichotillomania is a time-thief; there are many constructive and valuable ways to spend time doing things you like, or learning new hobbies. You know what your good at, practice your positive hobbies and feel joyful about your life.

Sabrina A. Kendall 2

Things to Avoid

1. Avoid looking too long at your hair or scalp in the mirror; this usually causes the hair pulling to start up.

2. Avoid becoming socially isolated, this can cause hair pulling episodes.

3. Avoid eating foods that causes constipation, which will assist in making the scalp itchy. For instance, frequent consumption of cheeses, chocolates, sugary snacks, etc., eat them in moderation.

4. Avoid friends that are a bad influence, negative people can have an affect on you in some way.

5. Avoid idle time, do things that will keep you busy and entertained until you're sleepy.

Do diligent activities such as house chores, long walks at a recreational park, spend time at a local library, crocheting, physical exercise, cooking family meals, doing a jigsaw puzzle with friends, and other fun positive activities.

30 Day Rehab Challenge for Trichotillomania 3

What is OCD Obsessive Compulsive Disorder?

OCD is an anxiety disorder that is characterized by unreasonable thoughts that lead to compulsive behavior. An Obsessive Compulsive Disorder causes the brain to continuously stay on a thought or urge.

OCD categories:

- Kleptomania - an obsessive impulse to steal regardless of financial need.
- Nymphomania - frequently preoccupied with sex.
- Counters - are obsessed with being organized and arranging things by order.
- Hoarders - compulsively hold on to things in fear that they might need them one day.
- Washers - afraid that their hands might get contaminated.
- Checkers - repeatedly check things like doors and stoves which associate them with feelings of harm and danger.
- Over eaters - excessive eaters that eventually leads to obesity.
- Trichotillomania - individuals that pull their own hair out of their head repeatedly.
- And other OCD behaviors. . . . .

Sabrina A. Kendall 4

Most individuals with OCD disorders are intelligent people and productive in other areas of their lives; they just have to tap into what they are good at and continue doing that.

Symptoms of Trichotillomania

People that pull their hair out of their scalp are commonly known for having repetitive awfulizing thoughts. Hopefully those obsessive thoughts can quickly switch to useful thoughts instead of destructive thoughts. Meditating on a pattern of bad thoughts can eventually lead to depression. This is when the hair-pulling habit has gotten worse, and might require medication from a medical doctor to treat the depression.

Trichotillomania is an attack on the mind, but it's still not a mental disorder. Although it will take a great amount of mind-renewing exercises and meditation to fight it until it's non-existent. I can say trichotillomania reminds of people that secretly smoke cigarettes and they won't to desperately stop. Except with cigarette smokers they might have to get their lungs checked by a doctor, and with pulling hair God gives us many chances because hair grows back about 1-2 ½ inches every month.

Like I've mentioned before, I've been pulling my hair out for 10 years. I'm not a medical doctor or a Psychiatrist, but I've been going through this trichotillomania fight off and on.

Sabrina A. Kendall 6

And now I want to help others that have trichotillomania, with the 30 day challenge that help me decrease bald spots due to hair pulling.

Most people such as myself would like to hear from people that actually been through the same things that others have, and learn how they deal with it to try and overcome it.

Symptoms - OCD behavior of compulsive hair pulling can eventually lead to:

- Permanent hair loss
- Depressive thoughts
- Carpal Tunnel Syndrome (hand to elbow pain)
- Avoiding windy outdoor weather
- Avoiding social events more often than usual
- Not accepting employment due to shame of bald spots
- Wearing wigs, weaves, scarves, and hats more often

I remember one year I had head congestion (headaches) and had to go to my doctor to get antihistamine pills, because I pulled so much hair out during that time. The outdoors wind would make my scalp cold, even though the hair weave I was wearing was supposed to cover the bald spots.

I never had sinus problems like that before until the trichotillomania. This is why the hair-pulling has to stop as soon as a person notices that they are forming bald spots, the sooner an individual gets help, the better.

Thank you for purchasing this book, you're on your way to overcoming trichotillomania, this is a huge step for you. My prayers go out to (God) our Father which is in Heaven about breaking the strong-hold of trichotillomania on everyone that reads this book.

It's always easy to start a habit and difficult to break a habit. Let's replace this awful habit with a therapeutic habit today. It's going to be a fight, so get ready mentally and spiritually to win this fight over your enemy (trichotillomania).

I read somewhere; a person admitted that hair-pulling felt good when they pulled their hair out. I decided not to let that thought transmit to my mind, because I know that everything that feels good is not good for me. There are times when hair pullers can go about 5 days without pulling, this gives us hope. The key is to stay busy doing things that keep your mind and hands moving for the sake of good.

Sabrina A. Kendall 8

Pulling hair while trying to sleep at night is pitiful, I can say that because I can relate. From the mouth of Joyce Myer (TV Pastor) "You can choose to be pitiful or powerful".

God has not given us a spirit of fear, but of power and of love and of a sound mind. 2 Timothy 1:7

Try and throw away the negative thoughts you've been having, by writing them down on paper and shredding the paper after you've read it. Now began to welcome into your mind the enthusiasm of recovery from trichotillomania by reading and putting into action new useful tools.

A good technique to use when going to sleep and prevent hair pulling is, count backwards from 100-1 (in your mind). I've counted in my mind many nights to prevent from pulling hair and loosing hours of sleep. Starting to count from 100 down to 1 helps you think harder on the numbers and less on the hair pulling. Also wear winter gloves to bed at night, and have someone tape the wrist-part of the gloves onto your wrist, apply the tape loosely.

We have to fight the urges and not let the urges be a giant over us. If God gives us the power to fight any bad habit, we have to be clever with it. Trichotillomania don't care about us, continuous hair-pulling is clever in its own ways.

30 Day Rehab Challenge for Trichotillomania 9

You have to be clever in ways of breaking the chains that bind you to pulling your own hair out.

Sabrina A. Kendall 10

OCD Quiz for Trichotillomania

1. Do you pull your hair out when you're tired or sleepy?
2. Do you write down the thoughts you're having when pulling hair?
3. Do you use devices to help you stop pulling hair?
4. What are the devices you use to help stop the hair-pulling (such as affirmations, Bible verses, positive music, learning a new hobby, etc.)?
5. Do you pull your hair out in public places?
6. Where are you, when you pull hair most of the time?
7. What time of day are you showing signs of trichotillomania?
8. Have you told a doctor that you need help with trichotillomania?
9. Do you wear wigs, weaves, hair extensions, scarves, or hats in public?
10. Have you exposed the fact that you have trichotillomania to a family member?
11. Will you ever tell a doctor or family member that you are in recovery of hair pulling?
12. How many years have you had trichotillomania?

30 Day Rehab Challenge for Trichotillomania 11

13. Are you employed full-time or part-time, or are you enrolled in school?

14. Do you have constructive (positive) hobbies that you do daily?

15. Which do you do when your scalp itches?

- Pull hair out in the area of the itchy scalp?
- Compulsively wash your scalp?
- Scratch the scalp without pulling in the area of the itch.
- Pick your skin in the area of the itchy scalp.
- Pat your head with your hand until the scalp stops itching.

16. Are you eating foods high in vitamin C and drinking 100% fruit drinks to prevent an itchy scalp?

17. If you pull hair out in the mornings do you change your behavior to doing something else instead of the trichotillomania, such as physical exercise, home chores, crocheting, etc.?

18. Do you have a journal (notebook) where you write down happy moments of your life, from the past to the present?

19. Did your hair fill-in during your last 30 day challenge?

20. Do you avoid gazing-off into the mirror at your hair, in preventing pulling strands of hair out?

Answer these same questions every month, on a blank paper by numbering the paper from 1-20.

Your Hair is Part of Your Beauty

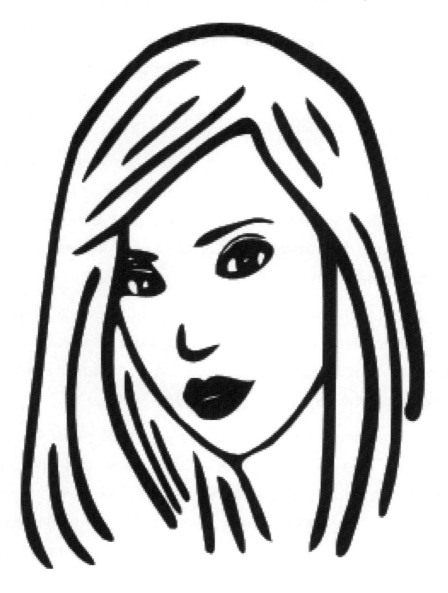

Sabrina A. Kendall 14

How to Stop Pulling Hair Out

First you can start your day by reading daily devotions or Bible verses. Giving God the first part of your day is acknowledging Him first, and not thinking about hair pulling in the morning.

When you eat breakfast, lunch, and dinner, ask in prayer to God for "healing" over your mind and body each time of day you have meals. Eventually the words of healing and the prayer will consume you instead of the trichotillomania impulses.

But when you do pull hair out, right down how long you've went without pulling. You can use a stop-watch or a timer on a cell phone to note how long you haven't pulled throughout the day.

Weaning yourself off of hair pulling is possible; it's going to take everything you've learned in this book. It might not take just one thing to stop the hair pulling, because every device works hand-in-hand. It will take everything possible to fight the thoughts and urges of trichotillomania.

30 Day Rehab Challenge for Trichotillomania 15

The Spirit in us is willing but the flesh is weak. This is why you have to stay encouraged and hopeful about stopping the urges. It's been said that it takes 21-30 straight days to break a bad habit. It may take some people longer than 30 straight days to prevent from relapse of repetitive trichotillomania behavior.

When you do catch yourself pulling hair out; place each pulled hairs on a white sheet of paper instead of putting the hair on the floor. This makes you very aware about the trichotillomania behavior. The reason for placing the pulled hairs on a white sheet of paper is to allow you to become more conscious of how many you've pulled out during each trance.

** I have an exercise for you to try; reach up to your head and hold a strand of hair for as long as possible without pulling it. Time yourself with a clock-timer for 3-5 minutes while holding the strand of hair, you can maybe rub the strand of hair but avoid pulling it. Do this same exercise every week to test your strength in avoid trichotillomania impulses. After you do this exercise, place strips of tape on your fingertips and put gloves on for as many hours as possible.

Sabrina A. Kendall 16

If I can decrease hair pulling episodes in a 30 day rehab challenge, you can too. I pray for your strength just as my Mom prayed for me.

Tape Your Fingertips Device

Try taping your finger tips with tape; of course avoid applying the tape tightly. Lightly apply tape to each fingertip to prevent from pulling your hair. Apply tape to your thumbs and pointer fingers first and immediately if you're in a trance of hair pulling in that moment. If you really want to go 30 days without pulling hair out, you will try the tape method. It's either continue hiding bald spots in your scalp, or have taped fingertips.

During my 30 day rehab challenge of trichotillomania, I had tape on my fingertips all through the day. I just kept reapplying the tape at every chance, and then putting gloves on over my hands while my fingertips were taped.

Wearing tape on your fingertips makes it hard to feel the strands of hair, especially when your not looking into the mirror at your scalp and hair for a long period of time.

After the 30 day challenge you will notice your hair getting thicker, and you will have no more bald spots when using this method of applying tape to your fingertips. You may have to apply the tape to the fingertips in a creative way, to make sure the tape is hanging over the fingertips and thumbs. Taping your fingertips may be one of your last things to exercise in stopping to pulling out your hair.

Sabrina A. Kendall 18

This is why it's crucial to be enthusiastic about trying the tips in this book, because it can help save you from the impulses of trichotillomania.

When you're ready to take the tape off your fingertips, began to wash your hands while the tape is still on with a lot of soap and warm water. The soapy hand washing will loosen-up the tape on the fingers and makes it easy for the tape to peel off. **Remember to peel the tape off slowly, to prevent from hurting your skin.**

But most of the day instead of taking the tape off, you can cleanse your hands with hand-sanitizer. Apply a scarf on your head when the tape is off the finger tips, until you can reapply the tape.

Reapply the tape after brushing teeth, eating, showering, and going to the bathroom. Get used to it; the tape will be on your fingers throughout the day. The tape will be on while you're on the computer; you may have to type with one finger though. The tape will be on while doing your hobbies such as learning to do embroidery (fun). And the tape will be on your finger-tips while sleeping at night as well.

30 Day Rehab Challenge for Trichotillomania 19

Your main goal for stopping the hair pulling would be "how bad do you want to stop this bad habit?" Most of the time you may have to think that you want to stop the hair-pulling so bad, that your life depends on it. You have to fantasize in your mind that you already don't pull hair out anymore and how great it makes you feel. If you want to be successful in overcoming trichotillomania you have to do what it takes to stop.

Expose the trichotillomania, don't let the trichotillomania expose you.

When applying hair products on your hair and scalp such as shampoo, oils, etc., call on healing from God to cast away the urges of hair pulling. Yes, it's going to take all that's possible to fight the trichotillomania giant. And one day you will look back after the rehabilitation stage and realize the trichotillomania wasn't that huge. At times people with negative habits need to be saved from their own self.

Sabrina A. Kendall 20

Claim Healing Over Your Body

I heard of a guy that prayed "healing" over his water and other liquids he drank. This is a great idea, it was said that the guy that prayed healing over his water began to have better health reports from his doctor.

Words are powerful; continue speaking healing over your mind and body, to eventually stop the pulling impulses. The Heavenly Father created the world with words, so words are powerful for humans as well. After all, we are made in the image of the Spirit of God. The more you read this book over and over again, it will begin to sound different each time. Faith comes by hearing, so it's important that you hear yourself reading books that will help with the hair-pulling behavior.

Listen to Gospel songs daily, that has the word "healing" in the title or in the lyrics. Read Bible verses daily that pertains to healing; the book of Matthew is a good source for healing scriptures.

30 Day Rehab Challenge for Trichotillomania 21

When you're getting ready for bed at night, play those "healing" Gospel songs in your mind while on your way to sleep.

What is it you want to do with your life, if you had no more bald spots and urges to pull hair?

Sabrina A. Kendall 22

30 Day Challenge

Start your 30 day challenge today and end it in 30 days. For instance, if today is the 10th day of the month, end your 30 day challenge on the 10th day of next month. Write on a calendar the words "start 30 day challenge," and write on the 30th day "the end of a 30 day challenge."

On the first day of the 30 day rehab challenge, take photos of your hair without any hair-extensions, and write the day, month, and year on the front of the photo. Take another photo of your hair on the 30th day of the challenge, and write the month, day, and year on it also. There should be results of progress in every 30 day challenge of decreased hair pulling episodes. There are people that have actually overcame trichotillomania, so it is possible to stop the pulling impulses. Just say to yourself, "I believe I will eventually stop pulling my hair out, it is possible."

With this 30 day challenge you may want to make a trichotillomania report card, and mark a grade A, B, C, D, or F. The letter A is for excellence meaning you didn't pull any hair on that day. But you would have to wait until the next day of course to grade your behavior of hair pulling for that previous day.

30 Day Rehab Challenge for Trichotillomania 23

This 30 day rehab challenge will consist of taping your finger tips for 30 days straight or more days if needed. Rehabilitation is part of recovery with trichotillomania behavior, and growing back hair where there were bald spots.

There will also be days that you may fall off and begin to pull hair out again after 7 days, 30 days, or longer than that. The challenge is to keep getting back up and continue to fight; this is how you exercise the strength you have for overcoming trichotillomania. You will become stronger and stronger the more times you put yourself on another 30 day challenge, if that's what it takes.

With women the urges to pull hair out is even more tempting during the monthly menstruation cycle. During a woman's monthly period, the scalp will itch often than usual. This is when you have to be aware to use the devices in this book to prevent from reaching up to pull hair, due to an itchy scalp.

Hobbies can be a huge part of the recovery process also; it helps to replace hair pulling with something constructive. If you already have hobbies, practice them to keep your hands busy.

Sabrina A. Kendall 24

You have to be enthusiastic about your hobbies; which will make you want to do the hobby more than the trichotillomania behavior. It's also fun to learn new hobbies, a hobby that you're excited about when you wake up in the mornings.

There are many hobbies to learn:

Crocheting
Jigsaw puzzles
Sewing clothes
Painting
Cooking
Karaoke (singing)
Badminton
Swimming
Bike riding
Skating
Embroidery
Arts and crafts
Volunteer (library, senior center, food-drive, etc.)

Your local crafts store will have many things that can give you ideas on what hobbies you may want to learn. I buy crafts at Michaels, Hobby Lobby, Wal-mart craft isles, JoAnn Fabrics and Crafts, and any other local stores that sell crafts.

30 Day Rehab Challenge for Trichotillomania 25

Most local colleges have dance class, music instrument class, and theater classes to keep you active and entertained.

There are people on TV that exposed the fact that they have trichotillomania. There was a lady on the Tyra Banks talk show, that has OCD trichotillomania and she said she pulls her hair out because her scalp itches all the time. **Remember when your scalp is itching that just means the hair is growing and the scalp is healing.**

Are your thought patterns a line of negative thoughts or a combination of both? We have to be conscious of when we have a pattern of negative thoughts, and begin to change the channel in our mind. To have a thought pattern of positive thoughts is really useful and it's possible in decreasing depression. Try and throw a birthday party for a family member, this will create a fun memory. Positive thoughts also come from fun memories and happy moments. Many people get their happy moments from family, friends, hobbies, TV shows, good food, good music, social events, etc.

How can the Holy Bible help with a speedy recovery of trichotillomania? Certain Bible verses can help cleanse us from any thing we are going through, you just have to find the right verses. People like reading Proverbs, Corinthians, James, Timothy, Psalm, Ephesians, Matthew, and many other books in the Holy Bible. The Bible is the world's best seller in books, it's not just a book, it's "The Book."

Success is difficult for many people without Christ as the foundation in their life; you will be successful in overcoming trichotillomania. Yes it will take small steps to eventually get to the finish line, but it is well worth it.

"Anything is possible to them that believe." Mark 9:23

If you believe within your heart; you will one day look back and say "I use to be a hairpuller and now I'm healed by the grace of God." It all starts with believing, you are already healed, just have to keep the faith and apply positive actions. Faith comes by hearing, and hearing by the word of God. So keep hearing the word of God and reading it, this bad habit you have will eventually pass. Let go of the guilt of hair pulling, God doesn't want us to go around feeling guilty. God wants you to have joy and not let anything take away your joy.

30 Day Rehab Challenge for Trichotillomania 27

Listen to Inspirational Music

Music can help us be in a happy state of mind or it can do the opposite. Inspirational music can uplift the spirit and prevent us from having depressive moods. Being consistent with listening to inspirational music is the idea, listen to it in the car, on a cell phone, mp3 player, computer, when taking a shower, etc.

Research has proven people that listen to rock music, heavy metal, and any other music that have negative or dark lyrics are more likely to eventually become depressed or suicidal. Music with uplifting positive lyrics will keep you in a joyful and lively mood. Try to have to a chain reaction of all things positive from music, books, environments, foods, TV shows, movies, the people we share time with, etc. The trichotillomania needs to be dealt with in every way possible.

When your singing along with the Gospel music, really try and feel it in your spirit. Begin to see yourself with no bald spots, allow the words of the Gospel song to cleanse your mind. In your mind begin to shake off the chains from your neck, ankles, and wrists; those chains have had you enslaved to pulling your long enough.

Sabrina A. Kendall 28

It's time to exercise your faith and live free of trichotillomania, by doing a 30 day rehab challenge to stop pulling your hair out.

Gospel music - is the good news and teachings of Christ the Messiah and the Apostles; the Christian revelation.

Develop a Daily Routine

Be consistent with a daily routine/schedule, avoid having idle time or down time. From the time you wake up in the morning until you lie down at night, write down a daily routine and stick to it. Acknowledge the days that you don't pull your hair, and write it down with a date next to it, example: 12/24/xxxx "I didn't pull my hair out yesterday, I was busy with a hobby, doing physical exercise, cooking a family meal, taking a long walk in the park, singing karaoke with friends, etc."

Some people that are Christians go on a fast, to help with bad habits. A fast is when there is prayer each day of the fast; reading Bible verses about healing, no eating just drinking water for a few days. Jesus Christ fasted 40 days and nights to prevent from being tempted by the devil.

Women are commonly known for having long hair, our hair is our beauty. Whereas most men can shave their heads if they have trichotillomania to prevent hair pulling urges. Statistics show that there are more women that have trichotillomania than men.

A full head of hair makes people look healthier and financially prosperous, but thinning hair with bald spots make people look sick and poor.

Sabrina A. Kendall 30

I know this because I have before and after pictures of myself pre-trichotillomania, during, and post-trichotillomania.

Avoid making yourself feel like a victim due the hair pulling, instead continue to find self-worth in your job, hobbies, your character, spirituality, talents, etc.

Also avoid worrying and turn that into prayer, because worrying causes depression and prayer changes things for the better. There is no one magical thing or medication that will stop hair pulling; every tool you've learned in this book should be exercised to make weak areas stronger. Speaking of exercise, it's a good idea to add physical exercise to your daily routine list; this gives you one more thing to do rather than pulling out your hair.

The reason I wrote this book is to help people with trichotillomania, to stop pulling their hair out and to focus on something productive. There are ways of being productive and avoiding idle time, such as a job, going on long walks at a recreational park, hobbies, visiting family members, joining a local college, etc. Every day can be a goal-setting day, make a vision-board of things you want to do and when you want them completed.

30 Day Rehab Challenge for Trichotillomania 31

If you belong to a Christian church, ask the Saints (elders) of the church to pray for your deliverance of trichotillomania. After pulling your own hair out, you have to try everything that can possibly stop the urges.

The difficult part is not the hair pulling, it's changing your mind to think of something new and engage in it. It's been said that one bad habit follows another bad habit. In this case we are going to let many good habits chase away the trichotillomania. As you already know, hair pulling keeps you out of balance. And God doesn't want His children to be out of balance in any area of life. When being out of balance other bad habits can creep in, that's why bad habits need to stop before they get worse. Anyone that has OCD is out of balance and in a struggle, but keep the hope, there is a way out. You have to forgive yourself for the bad habits and also for feeling guilty. Hold on to your joy because the joy of the Lord is your strength. (Nehemiah 8:9)

It's been said, if a person keeps doing the same thing and expect different results, they are senseless. But if you want different results, you have to stop doing the same thing you've been doing and do something different.

Sabrina A. Kendall 32

Self-Affirmations

Say to yourself in the mirror "I don't like pulling my hair" the more you say it every day; you will come out of the struggle of trichotillomania. Also say in the mirror, "I don't like the way it feels when I pull my hair out," "I hate the way it sounds when I pull my hair," and "I refuse to have bald spots on my head." Using ideas to help stop the hair pulling is like doing physical exercise; it has to be applied daily to eventually notice results. No one does physical exercise for 1 or 5 days and decides to stop exercising because they don't see results. Sometimes it takes 6 months, 1 year, or 5 years to see results of something you have been working at. Actually the work you put in to change your life for the better becomes a lifestyle.

Avoid situations, people, events, etc., that can trigger the urges to pull your hair out. In life we have to choose to be happy, no matter the situations going on around us. Forgiving people that has hurt you is not giving them power, but it's allowing you taking back your power. Live life for today and enjoy it to the fullest, because tomorrow isn't here yet, live in the moment and live today.

Say to yourself "I love myself and my hair and I want to keep it in my scalp."

30 Day Rehab Challenge for Trichotillomania 33

After you read this book with enthusiasm, you will need to read it a few times to stay on course.

Also try using image-therapy when anxiety tries to enter in, (close your eyes if possible) and think of a happy time in your life. Do this every day before bed as well; think of happy events in your life and play those images over again in your mind until it makes you smile.

One day soon before you know it, you will notice your hair looking healthier and thicker with no bald spots. Remember "No Guilt."

Eat foods high in vitamin C to help build up your immune system and stop the itchy scalp. Foods high in vitamin C: kiwi fruit, oranges and lemons, bell peppers, guavas, papayas, broccoli, cauliflower, strawberries, and kale/Collard greens.

Other affirmations to say to yourself:

- I can stop the negative obsessive thoughts.
- I will be enthusiastic about stopping the trichotillomania.
- I will avoid idle time and work on my hobbies.
- My hair is my beauty.
- I don't like pulling my hair out.
- I will keep my fingertips taped up, to prevent hair-pulling.
- I'm still healed regardless of the sudden urges of trichotillomania.
- I will become more sociable and outgoing.
- No more guilt but joy instead.
- This too shall pass.
- I look more beautiful without the bald spots.
- I don't like the bald spots.
- I will challenge myself for 30 days to apply the tools in this book.
- I will not quit on overcoming trichotillomania.
- I will not continue to slip into a hair-pulling trance.
- I will not pull hair out while reading this book.
- I will soon actually like how my own hair looks again.

Better days are ahead, and taking photos will be something to look forward to rather than not wanting to be in photos, due to the thinning hair, wigs, and other hair-pieces.

30 Day Rehab Challenge for Trichotillomania 35

Take pictures of your hair with the bald spots, and save them in a private folder on your computer with a password, include the dates and year. Look at those photos with the bald spots every week, stare at them and write down your thoughts of each photo. And put photos of yourself when you had a full head of your own hair on your computer screen, and anywhere else in your home or car that will help you look at those photos.

Again try playing board games, card games, and doing jigsaw puzzles every week to participate in socializing with others, (mark these game events on your calendar).

Hope is never giving up.

Check out - Tips to Trichotillomania Recovery
http://hubpages.com/hub/Trichotillomaniarecovery

Printed in Great Britain
by Amazon.co.uk, Ltd.,
Marston Gate.